LIVER GALLBLADDER CLEANSE BOOK

Elevate your vitality with this comprehensive guide to a healthier, toxin-free life.

DR EMILY THOMPSON

Printed in the United States of America.

First Edition: November 2023

TABLE OF CONTENT

INTRODUCTION 1

Unveiling the Vital Duo: Understanding the Liver and Gallbladder 1

The Fundamental Roles of The Liver And Gallbladder 1

Liver: 1

- Metabolic Powerhouse: 1
- Detoxification: 1
- Storage and Release: 1

Gallbladder: 2

- Bile Storage: 2
- Bile Secretion: 2
- Digestive Support: 2

Why A Cleanse Is Crucial for Overall Well-Being 4

Elimination of Toxins: 4

Improved Digestive Health: 4

Enhanced Energy Levels: 4

Balanced Weight Management: 5

Support for Organ Function: 5

Enhanced Mental Clarity: 5

Skin Health: 6

Balanced Mood and Emotional Well-being: 6

CHAPTER ONE 7

The Cleansing Power: Science Behind Liver-Gallbladder Detoxification 7

Scientific Principles Guiding a Successful Cleanse 7

Nutrient-Rich, Whole Foods: 7

Hydration: 7

Liver Support: 7

Fiber Intake: 8

Reduced Processed Foods: 8

Probiotics for Gut Health:...8

Limiting Sugar and Refined Carbohydrates:.....................8

Intermittent Fasting:...8

Exercise: 9

Adequate Sleep:..9

Mind-Body Practices:...9

Individualized Approach: 9

The Synergy of Foods, Herbs, and Practices In Detox Support **10**

1. Cruciferous Vegetables and Herbs:................................10

2. Hydration and Lemon Water:...10

3. Fiber-Rich Foods and Probiotics: 10

4. Herbal Teas and Detoxifying Herbs:...............................11

5. Dark Leafy Greens and Exercise: 11

6. Antioxidant-Rich Foods and Meditation: 11

7. Intermittent Fasting and Sleep: 11

8. Alkaline Foods and Deep Breathing:..............................12

9. Elimination of Processed Foods and Stress Reduction: ...12

CHAPTER TWO **13**

Nature's Remedies: Herbal Elixirs for Liver-Gallbladder Harmony...**13**

Comprehensive Guide to Herbal Remedies: Nurturing Health Naturally **13**

1. Understanding Herbal Remedies: 13

2. Popular Herbal Remedies: 13

3. Methods of Herbal Administration: 13

4. Choosing Quality Herbs: 14

5. Herbal Remedies for Common Ailments: 14

6. Herbal Remedies and Traditional Medicine: 14

7. Herbal Safety and Precautions: 15

8. Growing Your Herbal Garden: 15

9. Herbal Remedies for Long-Term Wellness:.................15

10. Integrating Herbal Remedies into Daily Life: 15

Harnessing Nature's Pharmacy for Effective Cleansing: A Holistic Approach To Wellness......................................**17**

1. Herbal Teas for Gentle Detox: 17

2.Cleansing Greens and Superfoods:.............................17

3. Citrus Fruits for Refreshing Cleanses: 17

4. Culinary Herbs for Digestive Harmony: 18

5. Detoxifying Roots and Tubers: 18

6. Ayurvedic Cleansing Herbs: 18

7. Mindful Practices for Cleansing:..................................18

8. Healing Waters and Hydration: 19

9. Seasonal Cleansing Rituals: 19

10. Customizing Your Cleansing Ritual:............................19

CHAPTER THREE..**21**

Nourishing Your Way to Health: Dietary Strategies for Liver-Gallbladder Wellness **21**

Curated Dietary Plans for Nourishing the Liver And Gallbladder **21**

1. Hydration for Detoxification: 21

2. Liver-Friendly Vegetables:...21

3. Healthy Fats for Gallbladder Support: 21

4. Lean Proteins: 22

5. Fiber-Rich Foods for Digestive Health: 22

6. Liver-Cleansing Herbs:..22

7. Citrus Fruits for Gallbladder Health: 22

8. Probiotics for Gut Health:...22

9. Herbal Teas for Digestion: 23

10. Mindful Eating Practices: 23

11. Customizing the Plan:...23

Superfoods and Mindful Eating for Transformative Cleansing **24**

1. Superfood Green Smoothie: 24

2. Quinoa and Avocado Bowl: 24

3. Turmeric-Ginger Infused Detox Water: 24

4. Berry and Chia Seed Pudding:..25

5. Baked Salmon with Lemon and Dill: 25

6. Dark Leafy Green Salad: 25

7. Detoxifying Herbal Tea Blend: 25

8. Mindful Meditation Before Meals:....................................26

9. Probiotic-Rich Greek Yogurt Parfait: 26

10. Herbal Infusion Before Bed: 26

11. Reflective Journaling:..26

CHAPTER FOUR **28**

Mind-Body Connection: Stress Reduction Techniques for Liver-Gallbladder Harmony **28**

Understanding Stress's Impact on Liver and Gallbladder Health **28**

1. The Stress Response and Liver Function:.............................28

2. Influence on Gallbladder Contractions: 28

3. Inflammation and Liver Health:..................................29

4. Insulin Resistance and Fatty Liver: 29

5. Gallstone Formation and Stress:.................................29

6. Altered Gut Microbiota and Liver: 29

7. Mind-Body Connection: 30

8. Managing Stress for Liver and Gallbladder Health:.........30

9. Professional Guidance:...30

Mindfulness Practices and Stress Reduction Techniques: Cultivating Calm in The Midst Of Modern Life 32

1. Mindful Breathing: 32

2. Body Scan Meditation: 32

3. Guided Imagery:..32

4. Mindful Walking: 33

5. Mindful Eating:...33

6. Progressive Muscle Relaxation (PMR): 33

7. Yoga and Tai Chi:...33

8. Mindful Journaling: 34

9. Breath Awareness in Stressful Moments:......................34

10. Digital Detox and Mindful Technology Use:...................34

CHAPTER FIVE 35

Recipes for Radiance: Culinary Creations to Support Liver-Gallbladder Cleansing...35

Expertly Crafted Recipes for Delicious and Healthful Cleansing 35

1. Green Detox Smoothie: 35

2. Quinoa and Veggie Buddha Bowl: 36

3. Detoxifying Turmeric-Ginger Tea:...37

4. Baked Salmon with Lemon and Herbs: 37

5. Berry and Kale Salad with Lemon Vinaigrette: 38

6. Cleansing Cucumber Avocado Salad:............................39

7. Detoxifying Beet and Carrot Juice: 40

8. Zucchini Noodles with Pesto and Cherry Tomatoes:.......41

9. Spicy Lentil Soup with Greens:..42

10. Detoxifying Green Tea Chia Pudding:..........................43

11. Detoxifying Cabbage and Apple Slaw:........................44

12. Spirulina and Pineapple Smoothie Bowl:.......................45

13. Cleansing Cauliflower Rice Stir-Fry:...............................46

14. Chilled Detox Watermelon Gazpacho:.........................47

15. Herb-Infused Detox Iced Tea: 48

16. Detoxifying Green Pea and Mint Soup:.........................49

17. Cleansing Citrus and Avocado Salad:..........................50

18. Herb-Roasted Sweet Potatoes: 51

19. Lemon Turmeric Detox Water:.......................................52

20. Mango and Spinach Detox Smoothie:..........................53

Culinary Delights that Promote Detoxification....................54

1. Detoxifying Green Smoothie Bowl: 54

2. Turmeric-Ginger Lentil Soup:..55

3. Detox Salad with Lemon-Tahini Dressing: 56

4. Cleansing Lemon-Herb Baked Cod:..............................57

5. Detoxifying Berry and Beet Smoothie: 57

6. Quinoa and Vegetable Buddha Bowl: 58

7. Detoxifying Cucumber-Mint Lemonade: 59

8. Rainbow Detox Salad with Ginger-Lime Dressing:...........59

9. Detoxifying Green Tea and Berry Smoothie:....................60

10. Spiced Roasted Chickpeas: 61

CHAPTER SIX 62

A Holistic Approach: Exercise and Lifestyle Strategies for Lasting Cleansing Benefits 62

Integrating Movement and Lifestyle Practices for a Holistic Cleanse 62

1. Morning Yoga and Stretching: 62

2. Daily Nature Walks: 63

3. Mindful Breathing Exercises: 63

4. Body Brushing: 64

5. Evening Restorative Yoga: 64

6. Hydration Rituals: 64

7. Digital Detox: 65

8. Journaling and Reflection: 65

9. Social Connection: 66

10. Quality Sleep Hygiene: 66

Holistic Approaches for Maintaining Liver and Gallbladder Health 67

1. Balanced Nutrition: 67

2. Hydration: 68

3. Herbal Support: 68

4. Regular Physical Activity: 68

5. Stress Management: 69

6. Avoidance of Toxins: 69

7. Moderate Alcohol Consumption: 70

8. Healthy Fats: 70

9. Regular Health Check-ups: 70

10. Mindful Eating: 71

CHAPTER SEVEN 73

The Journey Within: Personal Experiences and Success Stories 73

Real-Life Accounts of Individuals Undergoing the Cleanse 73

1. Name: Olivia Martinez 73

2. Name: Alex Johnson 73

3. Name: Jasmine Carter 74

4. Name: William Chen 74

5. Name: Emily Rodriguez 75

6. Maria Gonzalez - Elementary School Teacher.................75

7. Dr. Ahmed Khan - Emergency Room Physician 76

8. Sophie Williams - Marketing Executive 76

9. Carlos Rodriguez - Construction Worker....................76

10. Alicia Chang - IT Professional...........................77

11. Eduardo Martinez - Small Business Owner 77

Learn From Experiences, Challenges, and Triumphs 78

Experiences:...78

Challenges:..78

Triumphs: 79

Reflection:..79

Adaptability:..80

Continuous Improvement:......................................80

Chapter Eight 82

Troubleshooting the Cleanse: Common Questions and Expert Answers 82

Addressing Common Concerns About Liver-Gallbladder Cleansing 82

1. Safety Concerns:..82

2. Detox Symptoms: 83

3. Impact on Medications: 83

4. Nutrient Deficiency: 84

5. Effectiveness: 84

6. Frequency of Cleansing: 85

7. Dehydration Concerns: 85

8. Pregnancy and Nursing: 86

Expert Insights, Tips, and Troubleshooting Advice for Liver-Gallbladder Cleansing 87

1. Consultation with Healthcare Professionals: 87

2. Hydration and Electrolyte Balance: 88

3. Mindful and Gradual Approach: 88

4. Incorporate Liver-Supportive Herbs: 89

5. Balanced Nutrition: 89

6. Mind-Body Practices: 90

7. Monitoring Detox Symptoms: 90

8. Post-Cleanse Transition: 91

CHAPTER NINE 93

Your Roadmap to Sustainable Wellness: Post-Cleanse Maintenance and Beyond 93

Navigating The Post-Cleanse Phase with A Sustainable Wellness Roadmap 93

1. Gradual Reintroduction of Foods: 93

2. Maintain Hydration and Detox Support: 93

3. Mindful Eating Practices: 94

4. Regular Exercise Routine: 94

5. Stress Management Techniques: 95

6. Regular Health Check-ups: 95

7. Holistic Wellness Practices:..96

8. Cultivate a Supportive Community: 96

Daily Habits and Practices for Enduring Liver and Gallbladder Health..**98**

1. Hydration:...98

2. Balanced Nutrition: 98

3. Herbs and Supplements:...99

4. Mindful Eating: 99

5. Regular Exercise: 100

6. Stress Management: 100

7. Limit Alcohol Consumption:... 101

8. Regular Health Check-ups: 101

9. Cultivate a Positive Mindset: 102

Conclusion **103**

INTRODUCTION
UNVEILING THE VITAL DUO: UNDERSTANDING THE LIVER AND GALLBLADDER

The Fundamental Roles of The Liver And Gallbladder

The liver and gallbladder are vital organs in the human body, each playing distinct yet interconnected roles in maintaining overall health and well-being.

LIVER:

- **Metabolic Powerhouse:** The liver is a metabolic hub, involved in various crucial functions such as converting nutrients from the food we eat into energy. It plays a central role in carbohydrate, protein, and fat metabolism.

- **Detoxification:** One of the liver's primary responsibilities is detoxifying the blood by removing harmful substances, including toxins and drugs. It transforms these substances into water-soluble compounds that can be excreted from the body.

- **Storage and Release:** The liver acts as a storage facility for essential nutrients like glycogen, vitamins, and minerals. It releases these stored substances into the bloodstream when the body needs them.

GALLBLADDER:

- **Bile Storage:** The gallbladder is a small, pear-shaped organ that stores bile produced by the liver. Bile is essential for the digestion and absorption of fats in the small intestine.

- **Bile Secretion:** When we consume fatty foods, the gallbladder releases bile into the small intestine to emulsify fats, breaking them down into smaller particles for better absorption by the body.

- **Digestive Support:** The gallbladder's role in fat digestion is crucial for the absorption of fat-soluble vitamins (A, D, E, and K) and helps in overall nutrient assimilation.

Together, the liver and gallbladder form an intricate system that contributes to digestion, nutrient processing, and overall detoxification. Their proper functioning is essential for maintaining a balanced and healthy internal environment in the body.

Why A Cleanse Is Crucial for Overall Well-Being

A cleanse is crucial for overall well-being because it serves as a targeted and intentional effort to support the body's natural detoxification processes and promote optimal functioning. Here are key reasons why a cleanse is considered essential for well-being:

Elimination of Toxins:

- Over time, the body accumulates toxins from various sources, including environmental pollutants, processed foods, and stress. A cleanse helps eliminate these toxins, reducing the burden on organs like the liver and kidneys.

Improved Digestive Health:

- Cleansing programs often involve dietary changes that support digestive health. Removing processed foods and incorporating nutrient-dense, easily digestible foods can enhance the efficiency of the digestive system.

Enhanced Energy Levels:

- By eliminating toxins and supporting nutrient absorption, a cleanse can boost energy levels. When the body functions optimally, it can more efficiently convert nutrients into energy, reducing feelings of fatigue and lethargy.

Balanced Weight Management:

- Cleansing can contribute to weight management by breaking unhealthy eating patterns, reducing cravings for processed foods, and promoting the consumption of whole, nutrient-rich foods. This can lead to a more balanced and sustainable approach to weight.

Support for Organ Function:

- Organs like the liver, kidneys, and colon play crucial roles in detoxification. A cleanse provides an opportunity for these organs to rest and regenerate, improving their overall efficiency and longevity.

Enhanced Mental Clarity:

- The connection between the gut and the brain is well-established. A cleanse that focuses on nourishing the gut can positively impact mental clarity and cognitive function. Removing inflammatory foods may also alleviate brain fog.

- Toxins can manifest in the skin as acne, inflammation, or other skin conditions. Cleansing supports skin health by reducing the internal burden of toxins, leading to a clearer complexion.

Balanced Mood and Emotional Well-being:

- The gut-brain axis influences mood and emotional well-being. A cleanse that supports gut health may positively impact mental and emotional states, contributing to a more balanced and positive outlook.

In summary, a cleanse is crucial for overall well-being as it addresses the cumulative effects of modern lifestyles and promotes a healthier, more resilient body. By supporting the body's natural detoxification processes, a cleanse can contribute to improved energy, digestion, mental clarity, and long-term health.

CHAPTER ONE
THE CLEANSING POWER: SCIENCE BEHIND LIVER-GALLBLADDER DETOXIFICATION
Scientific Principles Guiding a Successful Cleanse

A successful cleanse is often guided by scientific principles that aim to optimize the body's natural detoxification processes. While specific cleanse methods may vary, the following scientific principles are commonly considered for an effective and evidence-based approach:

Nutrient-Rich, Whole Foods:

- Focus on a diet rich in fruits, vegetables, whole grains, and lean proteins. These foods provide essential nutrients that support the liver, kidneys, and other organs involved in detoxification.

Hydration:

- Adequate water intake is crucial for flushing out toxins through urine and supporting overall cellular function. Hydration also aids in maintaining optimal kidney function.

Liver Support:

- Include foods that support liver function, such as cruciferous vegetables (broccoli, cauliflower), beets, and antioxidant-rich foods. These substances assist the liver enzymes in the detoxification process.

Fiber Intake:

- Dietary fiber promotes regular bowel movements, aiding in the elimination of waste and toxins. Whole grains, legumes, and vegetables are excellent sources of fiber.

Reduced Processed Foods:

- Minimize the intake of processed foods, which often contain additives, preservatives, and artificial substances that may burden the body's detoxification pathways.

Probiotics for Gut Health:

- Probiotics support a healthy balance of gut bacteria, which plays a role in overall health and can influence the body's ability to eliminate toxins. Include fermented foods like yogurt, kefir, and sauerkraut.

Limiting Sugar and Refined Carbohydrates:

- Excessive sugar and refined carbohydrates can contribute to inflammation and disrupt the balance of gut bacteria. A cleanse often involves reducing these substances to support overall health.

Intermittent Fasting:

- Some cleansing approaches incorporate intermittent fasting, which allows the digestive system to rest and promotes autophagy – a cellular repair process that may aid in detoxification.

Exercise:

- Regular physical activity supports circulation, lymphatic drainage, and sweating, all of which contribute to the elimination of toxins from the body.

Adequate Sleep:

- Quality sleep is essential for overall well-being, including the body's ability to repair and regenerate. During sleep, the brain undergoes detoxification, clearing waste products.

Mind-Body Practices:

- Stress reduction through practices such as meditation, yoga, or deep breathing can positively impact the body's ability to detoxify. Chronic stress can hinder optimal organ function.

Individualized Approach:

- Recognize that individual responses to cleansing methods may vary. Factors such as age, health status, and medical history should be considered when designing a cleanse.

It's important to note that scientific evidence on the effectiveness of specific cleansing protocols can vary, and consulting with healthcare professionals before embarking on a cleanse is advisable, especially for individuals with underlying health conditions. A holistic and evidence-based approach ensures that a cleanse is both safe and beneficial for overall well-being.

The Synergy of Foods, Herbs, and Practices In Detox Support

The synergy of foods, herbs, and practices in detox support involves combining elements that work together to enhance the body's natural detoxification processes. Here's an exploration of how certain foods, herbs, and practices can synergistically contribute to effective detox support:

1. Cruciferous Vegetables and Herbs:

- **Foods:** Broccoli, kale, cabbage, Brussels sprouts.

- **Herbs:** Turmeric, cilantro.

- **Synergy:** Cruciferous vegetables contain compounds that support liver detoxification pathways. Turmeric, with its active compound curcumin, has anti-inflammatory properties, and cilantro may aid in heavy metal detoxification.

2. Hydration and Lemon Water:

- **Practices:** Adequate water intake, especially with lemon.

- **Synergy:** Hydration supports kidney function and overall detoxification. Lemon water provides vitamin C and may enhance the liver's ability to produce detoxification enzymes.

3. Fiber-Rich Foods and Probiotics:

- **Foods:** Whole grains, fruits, vegetables.

- **Practices:** Consumption of fermented foods.

- **Synergy:** Fiber promotes bowel regularity and waste elimination. Probiotics support gut health, influencing the balance of beneficial bacteria and aiding in the breakdown of toxins.

4. Herbal Teas and Detoxifying Herbs:

- **Herbs:** Dandelion, milk thistle, ginger.

- **Practices:** Herbal tea consumption.

- **Synergy:** Dandelion and milk thistle support liver function, while ginger has anti-inflammatory properties. Herbal teas can provide hydration and specific compounds that aid in detoxification.

5. Dark Leafy Greens and Exercise:

- **Foods:** Spinach, kale, Swiss chard.

- **Practices:** Regular exercise.

- **Synergy:** Dark leafy greens offer chlorophyll, which may support detoxification. Exercise enhances circulation, lymphatic drainage, and sweating, facilitating the elimination of toxins.

6. Antioxidant-Rich Foods and Meditation:

- **Foods:** Berries, dark chocolate, green tea.

- **Practices:** Mindfulness meditation.

- **Synergy:** Antioxidants in foods combat oxidative stress. Mindfulness practices like meditation can reduce stress, supporting overall well-being and aiding the body's detoxification.

7. Intermittent Fasting and Sleep:

- **Practices:** Intermittent fasting.

- **Practices:** Adequate sleep.

- **Synergy:** Intermittent fasting allows the digestive system to rest, promoting autophagy. Quality sleep supports overall health, including the body's repair and detoxification processes.

8. Alkaline Foods and Deep Breathing:

- **Foods:** Almonds, leafy greens, cucumber.

- **Practices:** Deep breathing exercises.

- **Synergy:** Alkaline foods may help balance the body's pH. Deep breathing supports relaxation and may enhance oxygenation, promoting optimal cellular function and detoxification.

9. Elimination of Processed Foods and Stress Reduction:

- **Practices:** Stress reduction techniques.

- **Foods:** Minimized processed foods.

- **Synergy:** Reducing stress and eliminating processed foods both contribute to a lower toxic burden on the body, supporting the effectiveness of detoxification processes.

By combining these elements, individuals can create a comprehensive approach to detox support that addresses various aspects of health, from liver function to gut health and overall well-being. As with any health-related practices, it's advisable to consult with healthcare professionals, especially for those with underlying health conditions.

CHAPTER TWO
NATURE'S REMEDIES: HERBAL ELIXIRS FOR LIVER-GALLBLADDER HARMONY

Comprehensive Guide to Herbal Remedies:

Nurturing Health Naturally

Herbal remedies have been an integral part of traditional medicine systems for centuries, offering natural solutions to promote health and well-being. This comprehensive guide explores the world of herbal remedies, providing insights into their uses, benefits, and considerations.

1. Understanding Herbal Remedies:

- **Definition:** Herbal remedies harness the therapeutic properties of plants for medicinal purposes.

- **Holistic Approach:** Herbs often provide a holistic approach, addressing the root cause of imbalances rather than just symptoms.

2. Popular Herbal Remedies:

- **Echinacea:** Boosts the immune system.

- **Ginger:** Relieves nausea and aids digestion.

- **Turmeric:** Anti-inflammatory and antioxidant properties.

- **Chamomile:** Calming and promotes sleep.

- **Peppermint:** Eases digestion and soothes headaches.

3. Methods of Herbal Administration:

- **Teas and Infusions:** Steeping herbs in hot water.

- **Tinctures:** Extracts in alcohol or glycerin.

- **Capsules and Tablets:** Convenient for standardized doses.
- **Topical Applications:** Balms, creams, and oils for skin conditions.

4. Choosing Quality Herbs:

- **Organic Sources:** Opt for herbs grown without synthetic pesticides.
- **Quality Extraction:** Choose reputable brands using proper extraction methods.
- **Research:** Understand potential interactions and contraindications.

5. Herbal Remedies for Common Ailments:

- **Digestive Issues:** Peppermint, ginger, fennel.
- **Stress and Anxiety:** Lavender, chamomile, passionflower.
- **Immune Support:** Elderberry, echinacea, astragalus.
- **Sleep Disturbances:** Valerian, passionflower, lemon balm.

6. Herbal Remedies and Traditional Medicine:

- **Ayurveda:** Indian traditional medicine uses herbs like ashwagandha and holy basil.
- **Traditional Chinese Medicine (TCM):** Ginseng, ginkgo, and licorice are staples.
- **Western Herbalism:** Utilizes herbs like St. John's Wort and milk thistle.

7. Herbal Safety and Precautions:

- **Consultation:** Seek advice from a qualified herbalist or healthcare professional.

- **Allergies and Sensitivities:** Be aware of potential allergic reactions.

- **Pregnancy and Medical Conditions:** Some herbs may be contraindicated.

8. Growing Your Herbal Garden:

- **Accessible Herbs:** Basil, mint, and chamomile are easy to grow.

- **Cultivation Tips:** Consider sunlight, soil, and watering needs.

- **Sustainable Harvesting:** Harvest herbs responsibly to support plant regeneration.

9. Herbal Remedies for Long-Term Wellness:

- **Adaptogens:** Herbs like ashwagandha and rhodiola help the body adapt to stress.

- **Daily Tonics:** Incorporate herbs like nettle or dandelion for ongoing health support.

- **Balancing Elixirs:** Create personalized herbal blends for specific health goals.

10. Integrating Herbal Remedies into Daily Life:

- **Culinary Herbs:** Incorporate herbs like garlic, rosemary, and thyme into cooking.

- **DIY Remedies:** Learn to make teas, tinctures, and salves at home.

- **Mindful Consumption:** Pay attention to how your body responds to herbal remedies.

This guide serves as a starting point for navigating the rich and diverse world of herbal remedies. While herbs can be powerful allies in promoting health, it's essential to approach their use with knowledge, respect, and an understanding of individual needs. Always consult with healthcare professionals, especially if you are pregnant, nursing, or have existing health conditions.

Harnessing Nature's Pharmacy for Effective Cleansing: A Holistic Approach To Wellness

Nature has endowed us with a rich pharmacy of plants and herbs, each possessing unique properties that can support the body's natural cleansing processes. This guide explores the synergy between nature's gifts and effective cleansing, providing insights into incorporating botanical remedies for a holistic approach to wellness.

1. Herbal Teas for Gentle Detox:

- **Dandelion Root Tea:** Supports liver function and aids digestion.
- **Nettle Tea:** Rich in nutrients, promotes kidney health.
- **Peppermint Tea:** Soothes the digestive tract and alleviates bloating.

2.Cleansing Greens and Superfoods:

- **Chlorella:** Binds to heavy metals and aids detoxification.
- **Spirulina:** Packed with nutrients, supports overall health.
- **Wheatgrass:** Cleanses the liver and boosts energy levels.

3. Citrus Fruits for Refreshing Cleanses:

- *Lemon:* Enhances liver function and alkalizes the body.
- *Grapefruit:* Supports digestion and metabolism.

- *Orange:* Rich in antioxidants, boosts immune function.

4. Culinary Herbs for Digestive Harmony:

- **Rosemary:** Stimulates digestion and has antioxidant properties.

- **Thyme:** Supports respiratory health and has antimicrobial properties.

- **Basil:** Anti-inflammatory and aids in digestion.

5. Detoxifying Roots and Tubers:

- **Ginger:** Anti-inflammatory, supports digestion.

- **Turmeric:** Powerful antioxidant, reduces inflammation.

- **Burdock Root:** Cleanses the blood and promotes skin health.

6. Ayurvedic Cleansing Herbs:

- **Triphala:** Balances the digestive system and detoxifies.

- **Ashwagandha:** Adaptogenic herb, supports overall well-being.

- **Trikatu (Ginger, Black Pepper, Long Pepper):** Aids digestion and metabolism.

7. Mindful Practices for Cleansing:

- **Yoga:** Twisting poses stimulate digestion and detoxification.

- **Meditation:** Reduces stress, supporting overall mental and physical well-being.

- *Deep Breathing:* Enhances oxygenation, promoting cellular detoxification.

8. Healing Waters and Hydration:

- *Cucumber-Infused Water:* Hydrates and supports kidney function.

- *Mint-Infused Water:* Refreshes and aids digestion.

- *Lemon and Ginger Detox Water:* Supports metabolism and liver health.

9. Seasonal Cleansing Rituals:

- *Spring Cleansing:* Emphasize bitter greens and liver-supportive herbs.

- *Summer Cooling:* Include hydrating fruits and herbs like cilantro.

- *Fall Harvest:* Focus on root vegetables and immune-boosting herbs.

10. Customizing Your Cleansing Ritual:

- *Listen to Your Body:* Pay attention to how different herbs and foods make you feel.

- *Gradual Changes:* Start with small adjustments and gradually incorporate more cleansing practices.

- *Consultation with Professionals:* Seek guidance from herbalists or healthcare providers for personalized advice.

By harnessing nature's pharmacy through these botanical remedies and practices, individuals can embark on a journey towards effective cleansing that nourishes both the body and the mind. As with any wellness approach, it's advisable to consult with healthcare professionals, especially for those with pre-existing health conditions.

CHAPTER THREE
NOURISHING YOUR WAY TO HEALTH: DIETARY STRATEGIES FOR LIVER-GALLBLADDER WELLNESS

Curated Dietary Plans for Nourishing the Liver And Gallbladder

Maintaining a well-balanced diet is essential for supporting the health of the liver and gallbladder. This curated dietary plan focuses on nourishing these vital organs through nutrient-rich foods and mindful eating practices.

1. Hydration for Detoxification:

- *Water:* Adequate hydration supports the liver in flushing out toxins. Aim for at least 8 glasses of water daily.

- *Lemon Water:* Add a splash of fresh lemon to water to enhance liver function and aid digestion.

2. Liver-Friendly Vegetables:

- *Leafy Greens:* Spinach, kale, and Swiss chard are rich in chlorophyll, supporting the liver's detoxification processes.

- *Cruciferous Vegetables:* Broccoli, cauliflower, and Brussels sprouts contain compounds that enhance liver function.

3. Healthy Fats for Gallbladder Support:

- *Avocado:* Provides monounsaturated fats, which are beneficial for gallbladder health.

- *Olive Oil:* Rich in antioxidants and supports the gallbladder in releasing bile for digestion.

4. Lean Proteins:

- *Fatty Fish:* Salmon, mackerel, and trout are high in omega-3 fatty acids, which promote liver health.

- *Lean Poultry:* Chicken and turkey provide protein without excessive saturated fats.

5. Fiber-Rich Foods for Digestive Health:

- *Whole Grains:* Quinoa, brown rice, and oats support digestive regularity.

- *Legumes:* Lentils, chickpeas, and black beans provide fiber and protein.

6. Liver-Cleansing Herbs:

- *Turmeric:* Contains curcumin, known for its anti-inflammatory and liver-protective properties.

- *Milk Thistle:* Supports liver function and regeneration.

7. Citrus Fruits for Gallbladder Health:

- *Grapefruit:* Assists in the breakdown of fats and supports gallbladder function.

- *Berries:* Rich in antioxidants, beneficial for overall health.

8. Probiotics for Gut Health:

- *Yogurt:* Contains probiotics that support a healthy gut microbiome.

- *Kimchi:* Fermented foods like kimchi promote gut balance and aid digestion.

9. Herbal Teas for Digestion:

- *Peppermint Tea:* Soothes the digestive tract and may alleviate gallbladder discomfort.

- *Dandelion Root Tea:* Supports liver function and promotes bile production.

10. Mindful Eating Practices:

- *Chew Food Thoroughly:* Adequate chewing aids digestion and nutrient absorption.

- *Regular Meal Times:* Establish a consistent eating schedule to support digestive rhythm.

- *Limit Processed Foods:* Reduce the intake of processed and fried foods that can strain the liver and gallbladder.

11. Customizing the Plan:

- *Individual Sensitivities:* Pay attention to how your body responds to different foods.

- *Consultation with Professionals:* Seek advice from a nutritionist or healthcare provider, especially if you have specific dietary needs or health concerns.

This curated dietary plan aims to provide a foundation for supporting the health of the liver and gallbladder. It's important to tailor the plan to individual preferences and needs, and consulting with healthcare professionals can ensure that it aligns with your overall well-being.

Superfoods and Mindful Eating for Transformative Cleansing

Embarking on a transformative cleansing journey involves not just the choice of foods but also adopting mindful eating practices. This curated plan integrates superfoods known for their cleansing properties with mindfulness techniques, creating a holistic approach to rejuvenate both the body and mind.

1. Superfood Green Smoothie:

- *Ingredients:* Spinach, kale, banana, chia seeds, and almond milk.
- *Benefits:* Packed with chlorophyll, antioxidants, and fiber for gentle detoxification.
- *Mindful Tip:* Sip slowly, savoring each nutrient-rich gulp.

2. Quinoa and Avocado Bowl:

- *Ingredients:* Quinoa, avocado, cherry tomatoes, cucumber, and lemon vinaigrette.
- *Benefits:* Quinoa provides protein, while avocado offers healthy fats for sustained energy.
- *Mindful Tip:* Chew deliberately, appreciating the textures and flavors.

3. Turmeric-Ginger Infused Detox Water:

- *Ingredients:* Sliced turmeric, ginger, lemon, and mint in water.
- *Benefits:* Turmeric and ginger have anti-inflammatory properties, aiding digestion.

- *Mindful Tip*: Take a moment to inhale the refreshing aroma before each sip.

4. Berry and Chia Seed Pudding:

- *Ingredients*: Mixed berries, chia seeds, almond milk, and a touch of honey.
- *Benefits*: Berries provide antioxidants, while chia seeds offer fiber for digestive health.
- *Mindful Tip*: Eat slowly, acknowledging the textures and natural sweetness.

5. Baked Salmon with Lemon and Dill:

- *Ingredients*: Wild-caught salmon, lemon, dill, and olive oil.
- *Benefits*: Salmon is rich in omega-3 fatty acids, supporting liver health.
- *Mindful Tip*: Engage all senses while savoring each bite.

6. Dark Leafy Green Salad:

- *Ingredients*: Mixed greens, beetroot, walnuts, and a balsamic vinaigrette.
- *Benefits*: Leafy greens and beets promote liver detoxification.
- *Mindful Tip*: Express gratitude for the nourishment before eating.

7. Detoxifying Herbal Tea Blend:

- *Ingredients*: Dandelion root, nettle, and chamomile.
- *Benefits*: Supports liver function and aids in relaxation.

- *Mindful Tip:* Embrace the warmth of the tea, focusing on each soothing sip.

8. Mindful Meditation Before Meals:

- *Practice:* Take a few minutes of mindful meditation before eating.

- *Benefits:* Reduces stress, enhancing digestion and nutrient absorption.

- *Mindful Tip:* Be present with the sensations of breath and the anticipation of the meal.

9. Probiotic-Rich Greek Yogurt Parfait:

- *Ingredients:* Greek yogurt, mixed berries, and a sprinkle of granola.

- *Benefits:* Supports gut health with probiotics and fiber.

- *Mindful Tip:* Eat with intention, acknowledging the nourishment provided.

10. Herbal Infusion Before Bed:

- *Ingredients:* Lavender, chamomile, and lemon balm.

- *Benefits:* Promotes relaxation and quality sleep.

- *Mindful Tip:* Sip slowly, allowing the calming herbs to prepare the body for rest.

11. Reflective Journaling:

- *Practice:* Journal thoughts and feelings about the day's nourishment.

- *Benefits:* Fosters awareness of the connection between food choices and overall well-being.

This curated plan combines the potency of superfoods with mindful eating practices, offering a transformative approach to cleansing. Adapt the plan to suit personal preferences and consult with healthcare professionals for personalized guidance on your wellness journey.

CHAPTER FOUR
MIND-BODY CONNECTION: STRESS REDUCTION TECHNIQUES FOR LIVER-GALLBLADDER HARMONY

Understanding Stress's Impact on Liver and Gallbladder Health

Stress, a ubiquitous element of modern life, can exert profound effects on the body, including the liver and gallbladder. This exploration delves into the intricate relationship between stress and these vital organs, shedding light on how chronic stress may impact their health.

1. The Stress Response and Liver Function:

- *Cortisol Release:* Stress triggers the release of cortisol, a hormone associated with the body's "fight or flight" response.

- *Impact on Glucose Production:* Elevated cortisol levels can stimulate the liver to produce more glucose, potentially contributing to insulin resistance over time.

2. Influence on Gallbladder Contractions:

- *Role of Cortisol:* Cortisol can affect the gallbladder by reducing the strength and frequency of contractions.

- *Impaired Bile Release:* Chronic stress may hinder the proper release of bile from the gallbladder, potentially leading to digestive issues.

3. Inflammation and Liver Health:

- *Inflammatory Response:* Prolonged stress can contribute to chronic inflammation, affecting liver health.

- *Impact on Liver Diseases:* Chronic stress has been linked to an increased risk of liver diseases, including non-alcoholic fatty liver disease (NAFLD).

4. Insulin Resistance and Fatty Liver:

- *Elevated Cortisol and Insulin Resistance:* High cortisol levels can contribute to insulin resistance, a condition associated with the development of fatty liver.

- *Accumulation of Fat:* Stress-induced insulin resistance may lead to the accumulation of fat in the liver.

5. Gallstone Formation and Stress:

- *Slowed Digestion:* Chronic stress can slow down digestion, potentially leading to gallstone formation due to reduced gallbladder contractions.

- *Influence on Cholesterol Levels:* Stress may impact cholesterol levels, a factor linked to gallstone development.

6. Altered Gut Microbiota and Liver:

- *Gut-Liver Axis:* Stress can alter the balance of the gut microbiota, influencing the gut-liver axis.

- *Impact on Liver Inflammation:* Changes in gut microbiota composition may contribute to liver inflammation and disease.

7. Mind-Body Connection:

- *Central Nervous System Influence:* The brain, through the central nervous system, communicates with the liver and gallbladder.

- *Stress Reduction Techniques:* Practices like meditation and deep breathing can positively influence the mind-body connection, potentially mitigating stress's impact.

8. Managing Stress for Liver and Gallbladder Health:

- *Mindfulness Practices:* Incorporate mindfulness techniques to reduce overall stress levels.

- *Regular Exercise:* Physical activity can be a powerful stress-reducer and supports both liver and gallbladder health.

- *Adequate Sleep:* Prioritize quality sleep, as it plays a crucial role in stress management and overall well-being.

9. Professional Guidance:

- *Consult Healthcare Professionals:* If stress is impacting your physical health, seek guidance from healthcare professionals.

- *Holistic Approach:* Consider a holistic approach that addresses both the psychological and physiological aspects of stress.

Understanding the intricate interplay between stress and liver-gallbladder health emphasizes the importance of adopting stress management strategies as part of a comprehensive approach to overall well-being. By nurturing mental and physical health, individuals can positively influence the health of these vital organs.

Mindfulness Practices and Stress Reduction Techniques: Cultivating Calm in The Midst Of Modern Life

In the hustle and bustle of modern life, incorporating mindfulness practices and stress reduction techniques is crucial for maintaining mental well-being. Explore the following strategies to foster a sense of calm, enhance resilience, and alleviate the impact of stress.

1. Mindful Breathing:

- *Technique:* Find a quiet space, sit comfortably, and focus on your breath. Inhale slowly, feel the breath filling your lungs, and exhale mindfully. Repeat for a few minutes.

- *Benefits:* Calms the nervous system, reduces anxiety, and promotes presence in the moment.

2. Body Scan Meditation:

- *Technique:* Lie down or sit comfortably. Bring attention to different parts of your body, starting from your toes to the top of your head. Notice any sensations without judgment.

- *Benefits:* Enhances body awareness, releases physical tension, and encourages relaxation.

3. Guided Imagery:

- *Technique:* Close your eyes and imagine a peaceful place, such as a beach or a forest. Engage your senses in the imagery, noting colors, sounds, and textures.

- *Benefits:* Shifts focus from stressors, induces relaxation, and promotes a positive mental state.

4. Mindful Walking:

- *Technique:* Take a slow, deliberate walk, paying attention to each step. Notice the sensation of your feet lifting, moving, and making contact with the ground.

- *Benefits:* Connects the mind and body, improves focus, and offers a refreshing break.

5. Mindful Eating:

- *Technique:* Engage all senses while eating. Notice the colors, textures, and flavors of your food. Chew slowly and savor each bite.

- *Benefits:* Enhances appreciation for food, aids digestion, and prevents overeating.

6. Progressive Muscle Relaxation (PMR):

- *Technique:* Tense and then gradually release different muscle groups, starting from your toes up to your head.

- *Benefits:* Reduces physical tension, promotes relaxation, and eases muscle stiffness.

7. Yoga and Tai Chi:

- *Technique:* Engage in gentle yoga or Tai Chi sequences, emphasizing breath awareness and mindful movement.

- *Benefits:* Combines physical activity with mindfulness, improves flexibility, and reduces stress.

8. Mindful Journaling:

- *Technique:* Write down your thoughts and feelings without judgment. Reflect on positive aspects of your day or express gratitude.

- *Benefits:* Promotes self-reflection, provides an outlet for emotions, and fosters a positive mindset.

9. Breath Awareness in Stressful Moments:

- *Technique:* During stressful situations, take a few moments to focus on your breath. Inhale deeply and exhale slowly to center yourself.

- *Benefits:* Interrupts the stress response, promotes clarity, and enables a more composed response to challenges.

10. Digital Detox and Mindful Technology Use:

- *Practice:* Designate specific times for technology use. Take breaks from screens to be present in the offline world.

- *Benefits:* Reduces information overload, improves focus, and minimizes stress associated with constant connectivity.

Incorporating these mindfulness practices and stress reduction techniques into your daily routine can contribute to a more balanced and resilient mindset. Experiment with different approaches to discover what resonates best with you, and remember that consistency is key to reaping the full benefits of these practices.

CHAPTER FIVE
RECIPES FOR RADIANCE: CULINARY CREATIONS TO SUPPORT LIVER-GALLBLADDER CLEANSING

Expertly Crafted Recipes for Delicious and Healthful Cleansing

Here are twenty expertly crafted recipes for delicious and healthy cleansing, complete with instructions and approximate nutritional information:

1. Green Detox Smoothie:

Ingredients:

- 1 cup kale leaves, stems removed
- 1/2 cucumber, peeled and sliced
- 1 green apple, cored and chopped
- 1/2 lemon, juiced
- 1 tablespoon chia seeds
- 1 cup coconut water
- Ice cubes (optional)

Instructions:

1. Place all ingredients in a blender.
2. Blend until smooth.
3. Add ice cubes if desired and blend again.
4. Pour into a glass and enjoy!

Nutritional Information:

- Calories: 180
- Protein: 4g
- Fiber: 10g
- Vitamin C: 60% DV
- Iron: 15% DV

2. Quinoa and Veggie Buddha Bowl:

Ingredients:

- 1 cup cooked quinoa
- 1 cup broccoli florets, steamed
- 1/2 cup shredded carrots
- 1/2 avocado, sliced
- 1/4 cup hummus
- Sprinkle of sesame seeds

Instructions:

1. Arrange cooked quinoa in a bowl.
2. Add steamed broccoli, shredded carrots, and sliced avocado.
3. Dollop hummus in the center.
4. Sprinkle sesame seeds on top.
5. Mix before eating for a delicious, nourishing bowl.

Nutritional Information:

- Calories: 420
- Protein: 15g

- Fiber: 12g

- Healthy Fats: 20g

Ingredients:

- 1 teaspoon ground turmeric

- 1 teaspoon grated ginger

- 1 tablespoon honey

- 1 lemon, juiced

- 2 cups hot water

Instructions:

1. Mix turmeric, ginger, honey, and lemon juice in a cup.

2. Pour hot water over the mixture.

3. Stir well and let it steep for 5 minutes.

4. Strain if desired and enjoy this soothing tea.

Nutritional Information:

- Calories: 40

- Antioxidants: Turmeric and ginger are potent antioxidants.

Ingredients:

- 2 salmon fillets

- 1 lemon, sliced

- 2 tablespoons olive oil

- 1 teaspoon dried thyme

- Salt and pepper to taste

Instructions:

1. Preheat oven to 375°F (190°C).

2. Place salmon fillets on a baking sheet.

3. Drizzle with olive oil, sprinkle thyme, salt, and pepper.

4. Top with lemon slices.

5. Bake for 15-20 minutes or until salmon flakes easily with a fork.

Nutritional Information:

- Calories: 350

- Protein: 30g

- Omega-3 Fatty Acids: 2.5g

5. Berry and Kale Salad with Lemon Vinaigrette:

Ingredients:

- 2 cups kale, chopped

- 1 cup mixed berries (strawberries, blueberries, raspberries)

- 1/4 cup feta cheese, crumbled

- 1/4 cup walnuts, chopped

- 2 tablespoons olive oil

- 1 tablespoon balsamic vinegar

- 1 tablespoon lemon juice

- Salt and pepper to taste

Instructions:

1. In a large bowl, combine kale, berries, feta, and walnuts.

2. In a small bowl, whisk together olive oil, balsamic vinegar, lemon juice, salt, and pepper.

3. Drizzle the dressing over the salad and toss gently.

4. Serve immediately and relish the vibrant flavors.

Nutritional Information:

- Calories: 320

- Fiber: 8g

- Vitamin C: 90% DV

- Calcium: 15% DV

6. Cleansing Cucumber Avocado Salad:

Ingredients:

- 2 cucumbers, spiralized or thinly sliced

- 1 ripe avocado, diced

- 1 cup cherry tomatoes, halved

- 1/4 cup red onion, thinly sliced

- Fresh cilantro, chopped

- Juice of 1 lime

- 1 tablespoon olive oil

- Salt and pepper to taste

Instructions:

1. In a large bowl, combine cucumber, avocado, cherry tomatoes, and red onion.

2. In a small bowl, whisk together lime juice, olive oil, salt, and pepper.

3. Drizzle the dressing over the salad, toss gently, and garnish with fresh cilantro.

Nutritional Information:

- Calories: 250

- Fiber: 10g

- Healthy Fats: 18g

- Vitamin K: 40% DV

7. Detoxifying Beet and Carrot Juice:

Ingredients:

- 2 beets, peeled and chopped

- 3 carrots, peeled and chopped

- 1 apple, cored and sliced

- 1-inch piece of ginger, peeled

- 1 lemon, peeled

- 2 cups water

- Ice cubes (optional)

Instructions:

1. In a blender, combine beets, carrots, apple, ginger, and lemon with water.
2. Blend until smooth.
3. Strain the juice to remove pulp if desired.
4. Pour into a glass over ice cubes and enjoy this vibrant detox elixir.

Nutritional Information:

- Calories: 120
- Vitamin A: 300% DV
- Vitamin C: 80% DV

8. Zucchini Noodles with Pesto and Cherry Tomatoes:

Ingredients:

- 2 large zucchinis, spiralized
- 1 cup cherry tomatoes, halved
- 1/4 cup pine nuts, toasted
- 1/2 cup fresh basil leaves
- 1/4 cup Parmesan cheese, grated
- 1 clove garlic
- 1/4 cup extra virgin olive oil
- Salt and pepper to taste

Instructions:

1. In a blender, combine basil, pine nuts, Parmesan, garlic, olive oil, salt, and pepper. Blend into a smooth pesto.

2. In a bowl, toss zucchini noodles with cherry tomatoes.

3. Drizzle pesto over the noodles and tomatoes, toss gently, and serve.

Nutritional Information:

- Calories: 280

- Protein: 8g

- Healthy Fats: 23g

9. Spicy Lentil Soup with Greens:

Ingredients:

- 1 cup dry lentils, rinsed

- 1 onion, diced

- 2 carrots, diced

- 2 celery stalks, diced

- 3 cloves garlic, minced

- 1 teaspoon cumin

- 1 teaspoon smoked paprika

- 1/2 teaspoon cayenne pepper

- 4 cups vegetable broth

- 2 cups kale, chopped

- Juice of 1 lemon

- Salt and pepper to taste

Instructions:

1. In a large pot, sauté onion, carrots, and celery until softened.

2. Add garlic, cumin, smoked paprika, and cayenne. Stir for 1-2 minutes.

3. Pour in vegetable broth and add lentils. Simmer until lentils are tender.

4. Stir in kale and cook until wilted.

5. Finish with lemon juice, salt, and pepper. Serve hot.

Nutritional Information:

- Calories: 350

- Protein: 18g

- Fiber: 15g

10. Detoxifying Green Tea Chia Pudding:

Ingredients:

- 2 green tea bags

- 1 cup hot water

- 1/4 cup chia seeds

- 1 tablespoon honey or maple syrup

- Fresh berries for topping

Instructions:

1. Steep green tea bags in hot water for 5 minutes. Remove the tea bags.

2. In a bowl, mix chia seeds with brewed green tea.

3. Stir in honey or maple syrup.

4. Refrigerate for at least 2 hours or overnight.

5. Top with fresh berries before serving.

Nutritional Information:

- Calories: 180

- Fiber: 12g

- Antioxidants: Green tea is rich in antioxidants.

11. Detoxifying Cabbage and Apple Slaw:

Ingredients:

- 2 cups shredded green cabbage

- 1 green apple, julienned

- 1/4 cup shredded carrots

- 1/4 cup fresh parsley, chopped

- 1 tablespoon apple cider vinegar

- 1 tablespoon olive oil

- 1 teaspoon Dijon mustard

- Salt and pepper to taste

Instructions:

1. In a large bowl, combine cabbage, apple, carrots, and parsley.

2. In a small bowl, whisk together apple cider vinegar, olive oil, Dijon mustard, salt, and pepper.

3. Pour the dressing over the slaw, toss gently, and let it sit for a few minutes before serving.

Nutritional Information:

- Calories: 120
- Fiber: 5g
- Vitamin C: 30% DV

12. Spirulina and Pineapple Smoothie Bowl:

Ingredients:

- 1 frozen banana
- 1/2 cup pineapple chunks
- 1 tablespoon spirulina powder
- 1/2 cup coconut water
- Toppings: sliced kiwi, chia seeds, granola

Instructions:

1. Blend banana, pineapple, spirulina, and coconut water until smooth.
2. Pour the smoothie into a bowl.
3. Top with sliced kiwi, chia seeds, and granola for added texture and nutrients.

Nutritional Information:

- Calories: 280
- Protein: 6g
- Iron: 15% DV

Ingredients:

- 2 cups cauliflower rice
- 1 cup broccoli florets
- 1 bell pepper, sliced
- 1 cup snap peas, trimmed
- 2 tablespoons low-sodium soy sauce
- 1 tablespoon sesame oil
- 1 teaspoon ginger, minced
- 2 cloves garlic, minced

Instructions:

1. In a wok or large pan, heat sesame oil over medium-high heat.
2. Add ginger and garlic, sauté until fragrant.
3. Add cauliflower rice, broccoli, bell pepper, and snap peas. Stir-fry until vegetables are tender-crisp.
4. Drizzle soy sauce over the stir-fry, toss to combine, and cook for an additional 2 minutes.

Nutritional Information:

- Calories: 180
- Fiber: 8g
- Vitamin C: 120% DV

14. Chilled Detox Watermelon Gazpacho:

Ingredients:

- 4 cups seedless watermelon, diced
- 1 cucumber, peeled and diced
- 1 red bell pepper, diced
- 1/4 cup red onion, finely chopped
- 2 tablespoons fresh mint, chopped
- 3 tablespoons lime juice
- Salt and black pepper to taste

Instructions:

1. In a blender, combine watermelon, cucumber, bell pepper, red onion, mint, and lime juice.
2. Blend until smooth.
3. Season with salt and black pepper to taste.
4. Chill in the refrigerator for at least 1 hour before serving.

Nutritional Information:

- Calories: 90
- Vitamin A: 50% DV
- Hydration: Watermelon is over 90% water.

Ingredients:

- 4 green tea bags
- 1 tablespoon fresh mint leaves
- 1 tablespoon fresh basil leaves
- 1 tablespoon honey or agave syrup
- 1 lemon, sliced
- Ice cubes

Instructions:

1. Steep green tea bags in hot water for 3-5 minutes. Remove the tea bags.
2. Add mint and basil leaves to the hot tea, let it cool to room temperature, and then refrigerate.
3. Once chilled, sweeten with honey or agave syrup.
4. Serve over ice with lemon slices.

Nutritional Information:

- Calories: 20
- Antioxidants: Green tea, mint, and basil are rich in antioxidants.

Ingredients:

- 2 cups frozen green peas
- 1 onion, chopped
- 2 cloves garlic, minced
- 1 potato, peeled and diced
- 4 cups vegetable broth
- 1/4 cup fresh mint leaves
- Juice of 1 lime
- Salt and pepper to taste

Instructions:

1. In a pot, sauté onion and garlic until softened.
2. Add green peas, potato, and vegetable broth. Simmer until vegetables are tender.
3. Blend the mixture with mint leaves until smooth.
4. Return to the pot, add lime juice, and season with salt and pepper.

Nutritional Information:

- Calories: 180
- Protein: 8g
- Fiber: 10g

17. Cleansing Citrus and Avocado Salad:

Ingredients:

- 2 oranges, peeled and sliced
- 1 grapefruit, peeled and segmented
- 1 avocado, sliced
- 2 cups mixed greens
- 1 tablespoon olive oil
- 1 tablespoon balsamic vinegar
- 1 teaspoon honey
- Salt and pepper to taste

Instructions:

1. Arrange oranges, grapefruit, avocado, and mixed greens on a plate.
2. In a small bowl, whisk together olive oil, balsamic vinegar, honey, salt, and pepper.
3. Drizzle the dressing over the salad and serve immediately.

Nutritional Information:

- Calories: 280
- Fiber: 10g
- Healthy Fats: 15g

Ingredients:

- 2 sweet potatoes, peeled and cubed
- 2 tablespoons olive oil
- 1 teaspoon dried rosemary
- 1 teaspoon dried thyme
- 1 teaspoon smoked paprika
- Salt and pepper to taste

Instructions:

1. Preheat oven to 400°F (200°C).
2. In a bowl, toss sweet potatoes with olive oil, rosemary, thyme, paprika, salt, and pepper.
3. Spread on a baking sheet in a single layer.
4. Roast for 25-30 minutes or until golden and tender.

Nutritional Information:

- Calories: 200
- Fiber: 6g
- Vitamin A: 400% DV

19. Lemon Turmeric Detox Water:

Ingredients:

- 1 lemon, sliced
- 1 teaspoon ground turmeric
- 1 teaspoon grated ginger
- 2 cups water
- Ice cubes (optional)

Instructions:

1. Fill a jug with water and add lemon slices, turmeric, and ginger.
2. Refrigerate for at least 1 hour to allow flavors to infuse.
3. Serve over ice cubes if desired.

Nutritional Information:

- Calories: 10
- Antioxidants: Lemon, turmeric, and ginger are rich in antioxidants.

20. Mango and Spinach Detox Smoothie:

Ingredients:

- 1 cup frozen mango chunks
- 1 cup spinach leaves
- 1/2 banana
- 1 tablespoon chia seeds
- 1 cup coconut water
- Ice cubes (optional)

Instructions:

1. Blend mango, spinach, banana, chia seeds, and coconut water until smooth.
2. Add ice cubes if desired and blend again.
3. Pour into a glass and enjoy this refreshing smoothie.

Nutritional Information:

- Calories: 220
- Protein: 6g
- Fiber: 8g

These recipes are not only delicious but also designed to promote a healthy cleansing process. Adjust portion sizes to meet your dietary needs and consult with a nutritionist if you have specific health concerns. Enjoy the nourishing and flavorful journey towards well-being!

Culinary Delights that Promote Detoxification

Embarking on a culinary journey that promotes detoxification involves incorporating nutrient-dense foods known for their cleansing properties. Here's a delightful selection of culinary creations designed to support the body's natural detox processes:

1. Detoxifying Green Smoothie Bowl:

Ingredients:

- 1 cup kale leaves, stems removed
- 1/2 cucumber, peeled and sliced
- 1 green apple, cored and chopped
- 1/2 lemon, juiced
- 1 tablespoon chia seeds
- 1 cup coconut water
- Toppings: Fresh berries, sliced kiwi, and a sprinkle of granola

Instructions:

1. Blend kale, cucumber, apple, lemon juice, chia seeds, and coconut water until smooth.
2. Pour into a bowl and arrange toppings for added texture and nutrients.

2. Turmeric-Ginger Lentil Soup:

Ingredients:

- 1 cup dry lentils, rinsed
- 1 onion, diced
- 2 carrots, diced
- 2 cloves garlic, minced
- 1 tablespoon turmeric powder
- 1-inch piece of ginger, grated
- 6 cups vegetable broth
- Fresh cilantro for garnish

Instructions:

1. In a pot, sauté onion, carrots, and garlic until softened.
2. Add turmeric and ginger, stirring for 1-2 minutes.
3. Pour in vegetable broth and add lentils. Simmer until lentils are tender.
4. Garnish with fresh cilantro before serving.

3. Detox Salad with Lemon-Tahini Dressing:

Ingredients:

- Mixed greens (kale, spinach, arugula)
- 1 cup cherry tomatoes, halved
- 1 cucumber, sliced
- 1/4 cup red onion, thinly sliced
- 1/3 cup chickpeas, cooked
- Dressing: 2 tablespoons tahini, juice of 1 lemon, 1 tablespoon olive oil, salt, and pepper

Instructions:

1. Toss mixed greens, cherry tomatoes, cucumber, red onion, and chickpeas in a bowl.

2. In a separate bowl, whisk together tahini, lemon juice, olive oil, salt, and pepper.

3. Drizzle the dressing over the salad and toss gently.

Ingredients:

- 2 cod fillets
- 1 lemon, sliced
- 2 tablespoons fresh dill, chopped
- 2 tablespoons fresh parsley, chopped
- 1 tablespoon olive oil
- Salt and pepper to taste

Instructions:

1. Preheat oven to 375°F (190°C).
2. Place cod fillets on a baking sheet.
3. Arrange lemon slices on top, sprinkle with dill and parsley, and drizzle with olive oil.
4. Season with salt and pepper.
5. Bake for 15-20 minutes or until fish is cooked through.

Ingredients:

- 1/2 cup mixed berries (strawberries, blueberries, raspberries)
- 1 small beet, peeled and chopped
- 1/2 banana
- 1 tablespoon flaxseeds
- 1 cup almond milk
- Ice cubes (optional)

Instructions:

1. Blend berries, beet, banana, flaxseeds, and almond milk until smooth.

2. Add ice cubes if desired and blend again.

3. Pour into a glass and enjoy the vibrant flavors.

6. Quinoa and Vegetable Buddha Bowl:

Ingredients:

- 1 cup cooked quinoa

- Mixed vegetables (broccoli, carrots, bell peppers)

- 1/2 avocado, sliced

- 1/4 cup hummus

- Fresh herbs (cilantro or parsley)

- Lemon-tahini dressing: 2 tablespoons tahini, juice of 1 lemon, 1 tablespoon olive oil, salt, and pepper

Instructions:

1. Arrange cooked quinoa in a bowl.

2. Add steamed or roasted mixed vegetables.

3. Top with avocado slices, hummus, and fresh herbs.

4. Drizzle with lemon-tahini dressing.

7. Detoxifying Cucumber-Mint Lemonade:

Ingredients:

- 1 cucumber, sliced
- Handful of fresh mint leaves
- Juice of 2 lemons
- 1-2 tablespoons honey or agave syrup
- 4 cups water
- Ice cubes

Instructions:

1. In a pitcher, combine cucumber slices and mint leaves.
2. Squeeze the juice of lemons into the pitcher.
3. Add honey or agave syrup and water.
4. Stir well and refrigerate for at least 1 hour.
5. Serve over ice cubes.

8. Rainbow Detox Salad with Ginger-Lime Dressing:

Ingredients:

- Kale or spinach leaves
- Shredded red cabbage
- Grated carrots
- Sliced bell peppers (red, yellow, or orange)
- Cherry tomatoes, halved
- Cucumber, sliced
- Sesame seeds for garnish

- Dressing: 1 tablespoon grated ginger, juice of 1 lime, 2 tablespoons soy sauce, 1 tablespoon sesame oil

Instructions:

1. In a large bowl, combine kale or spinach, red cabbage, carrots, bell peppers, tomatoes, and cucumber.

2. In a small bowl, whisk together ginger, lime juice, soy sauce, and sesame oil.

3. Drizzle the dressing over the salad and toss gently.

4. Sprinkle sesame seeds on top for extra crunch.

9. Detoxifying Green Tea and Berry Smoothie:

Ingredients:

- 1 cup brewed green tea, cooled

- 1/2 cup mixed berries (blueberries, raspberries, strawberries)

- 1/2 banana

- Handful of spinach leaves

- 1 tablespoon chia seeds

- Ice cubes

Instructions:

1. Blend green tea, mixed berries, banana, spinach, and chia seeds until smooth.

2. Add ice cubes if desired and blend again.

3. Pour into a glass and enjoy the antioxidant-rich smoothie.

Ingredients:

- 1 can chickpeas, drained and rinsed
- 1 tablespoon olive oil
- 1 teaspoon cumin
- 1/2 teaspoon paprika
- 1/2 teaspoon garlic powder
- Salt and pepper to taste

Instructions:

1. Preheat oven to 400°F (200°C).
2. In a bowl, toss chickpeas with olive oil, cumin, paprika, garlic powder, salt, and pepper.
3. Spread the chickpeas on a baking sheet in a single layer.
4. Roast for 20-25 minutes or until golden and crispy.
5. Allow to cool and enjoy as a crunchy, detoxifying snack.

These culinary delights not only tantalize the taste buds but also provide an array of nutrients and antioxidants to support your body's natural detoxification processes. As with any dietary changes, it's essential to listen to your body and consult with a healthcare professional or nutritionist if you have specific health concerns. Enjoy the nourishing and cleansing experience!

A HOLISTIC APPROACH: EXERCISE AND LIFESTYLE STRATEGIES FOR LASTING CLEANSING BENEFITS

Integrating Movement and Lifestyle Practices for a Holistic Cleanse

Embarking on a cleanse involves not only nourishing your body with wholesome foods but also incorporating mindful movement and lifestyle practices. This holistic approach supports overall well-being and enhances the effectiveness of the cleanse. Here are ways to integrate movement and lifestyle practices into your cleansing journey:

1. Morning Yoga and Stretching:

Practice:

- Begin your day with a gentle yoga session or stretching routine.
- Focus on movements that promote flexibility, balance, and increased blood flow.

Benefits:

- Enhances circulation, reduces stiffness, and sets a positive tone for the day.
- Encourages mindfulness and connection with your body.

Practice:

- Incorporate daily walks in natural surroundings, such as parks or trails.
- Aim for at least 30 minutes of moderate-paced walking.

Benefits:

- Boosts mood and reduces stress.
- Supports the body's natural detox processes by promoting lymphatic circulation.

Practice:

- Set aside a few minutes each day for mindful breathing exercises.
- Practice deep breathing or meditation to calm the mind.

Benefits:

- Reduces stress and supports mental clarity.
- Enhances relaxation, complementing the cleansing process.

4. Body Brushing:

Practice:

- Before your daily shower, use a natural bristle brush to gently exfoliate your skin.

- Brush towards the heart in circular motions.

Benefits:

- Stimulates the lymphatic system, aiding in detoxification.

- Improves skin health and promotes a sense of invigoration.

5. Evening Restorative Yoga:

Practice:

- Wind down in the evening with restorative yoga poses.

- Focus on postures that encourage relaxation and release tension.

Benefits:

- Supports better sleep quality.

- Facilitates digestion and aids in the body's repair processes during sleep.

6. Hydration Rituals:

Practice:

- Establish mindful hydration habits by starting your day with warm lemon water.

- Throughout the day, sip on herbal teas or infused water with cucumber and mint.

Benefits:

- Supports hydration, which is crucial for detoxification.
- Lemon water aids digestion and provides a refreshing start.

7. Digital Detox:

Practice:

- Designate specific times for technology use.
- Implement a digital detox period before bedtime.

Benefits:

- Reduces screen-related stress and improves sleep quality.
- Enhances relaxation and mental clarity.

8. Journaling and Reflection:

Practice:

- Dedicate time for journaling to reflect on your cleansing journey.
- Write down your thoughts, feelings, and any observations.

Benefits:

- Promotes self-awareness and mindfulness.

- Provides an outlet for emotional expression during the cleansing process.

9. Social Connection:

Practice:

- Foster positive social connections.
- Engage in activities with friends or family that bring joy and laughter.

Benefits:

- Supports emotional well-being and reduces feelings of isolation.
- Enhances overall mental and emotional resilience.

10. Quality Sleep Hygiene:

Practice:

- Establish a consistent sleep routine, aiming for 7-8 hours of quality sleep.
- Create a calming bedtime ritual to signal your body it's time to wind down.

Benefits:

- Supports the body's natural detoxification processes during sleep.
- Enhances overall energy levels and mental clarity.

By integrating these movement and lifestyle practices into your cleanse, you create a holistic approach that nurtures not only your physical health but also your mental and emotional well-being. Listen to your body, and tailor these practices to suit your individual preferences and needs. Always consult with healthcare professionals or fitness experts if you have specific health concerns or conditions. Enjoy the journey to a rejuvenated and balanced self!

Holistic Approaches for Maintaining Liver and Gallbladder Health

Maintaining liver and gallbladder health involves adopting holistic approaches that address various aspects of well-being. Here are holistic strategies to support the health of these vital organs:

1. Balanced Nutrition:

Approach:

- Prioritize a diet rich in fruits, vegetables, whole grains, and lean proteins.

- Include foods known for liver support, such as leafy greens, beets, carrots, and fatty fish.

- Opt for a variety of colors and textures to ensure a spectrum of nutrients.

Benefits:

- Provides essential nutrients for liver function.

- Supports bile production and aids gallbladder health.

2. Hydration:

Approach:

- Ensure adequate daily water intake.
- Incorporate hydrating foods like watermelon, cucumber, and celery.

Benefits:

- Supports digestion and the elimination of toxins.
- Maintains the viscosity of bile for optimal gallbladder function.

3. Herbal Support:

Approach:

- Explore herbs with known liver-protective properties, such as milk thistle, dandelion, and turmeric.
- Consider herbal teas like peppermint or chamomile for digestive support.

Benefits:

- Enhances liver detoxification pathways.
- Aids in gallbladder function and digestive comfort.

4. Regular Physical Activity:

Approach:

- Engage in regular exercise, including both cardiovascular and strength training.

- Aim for at least 150 minutes of moderate-intensity exercise per week.

Benefits:

- Promotes overall metabolic health.
- Supports blood flow to the liver and encourages bile production.

5. Stress Management:

Approach:

- Practice stress-reducing techniques such as meditation, deep breathing, or yoga.
- Prioritize sufficient rest and quality sleep.

Benefits:

- Reduces cortisol levels, which can impact liver health.
- Supports overall well-being and healthy digestion.

6. Avoidance of Toxins:

Approach:

- Minimize exposure to environmental toxins and pollutants.
- Choose organic produce when possible to reduce pesticide intake.

Benefits:

- Lessens the burden on the liver to process toxins.
- Supports the liver's natural detoxification capabilities.

7. Moderate Alcohol Consumption:

Approach:

- If consuming alcohol, do so in moderation.

- Consider alcohol-free days to allow the liver time for recovery.

Benefits:

- Reduces the risk of alcoholic liver disease.

- Supports gallbladder function by avoiding excessive demands.

8. Healthy Fats:

Approach:

- Include sources of healthy fats, such as avocados, nuts, and olive oil.

- Limit saturated and trans fats found in processed and fried foods.

Benefits:

- Supports the formation and release of bile.

- Encourages the metabolism of fats by the liver.

9. Regular Health Check-ups:

Approach:

- Schedule regular check-ups with your healthcare provider.

- Monitor liver enzymes and address any concerns promptly.

Benefits:

- Early detection of liver or gallbladder issues.
- Allows for timely intervention and lifestyle adjustments.

Approach:

- Practice mindful eating, paying attention to hunger and fullness cues.
- Chew food thoroughly to aid digestion.

Benefits:

- Supports healthy digestion and nutrient absorption.
- Prevents overloading the digestive system, including the gallbladder.

By embracing these holistic approaches, you create a supportive environment for liver and gallbladder health. It's essential to personalize these strategies based on individual needs and consult with healthcare professionals for personalized guidance. A holistic approach not only targets specific organs but promotes overall well-being, fostering a harmonious balance in the body.

Real-Life Accounts of Individuals Undergoing the Cleanse

1. Name: Olivia Martinez

Location: California

Occupation: Yoga Instructor

Age: 32

Olivia, a vibrant yoga instructor from sunny California, embarked on a cleanse to align her body and mind. Fueled by her passion for holistic well-being, she incorporated cleansing practices into her routine. With the Pacific breeze as her backdrop, Olivia embraced mindful movement, nourishing foods, and herbal remedies. The cleanse not only revitalized her energy but inspired her yoga students on a path to wellness.

2. Name: Alex Johnson

Location: New York

Occupation: Financial Analyst

Age: 40

In the bustling streets of New York, Alex, a dedicated financial analyst, sought a reset for both body and mind. Tackling stress and long work hours, he committed to a cleanse that combined nutritious meals and stress-relieving practices. Green smoothies became his go-to in the concrete jungle, fostering a newfound balance. The cleanse not only supported his liver and gallbladder health but also became a catalyst for a more mindful, healthier lifestyle.

3. Name: Jasmine Carter

Location: Texas

Occupation: Chef

Age: 28

Jasmine, a talented chef in the heart of Texas, recognized the need to detoxify her body from culinary indulgences. In her kitchen, she curated cleansing recipes, incorporating herbs and spices to enhance flavors. As she explored the synergy of foods in her Texan haven, Jasmine discovered that cleansing wasn't just a physical journey but a flavorful exploration that ignited her culinary creativity.

4. Name: William Chen

Location: Illinois

Occupation: Software Engineer

Age: 35

Amidst the tech landscape of Illinois, William, a dedicated software engineer, embraced a cleanse to counterbalance his sedentary work life. Integrating movement into his routine, he opted for weekend hikes and detoxifying herbal teas. The cleanse became a source of mental clarity, fostering innovative thinking in the world of algorithms. William's journey highlighted the importance of a holistic approach for professionals in the fast-paced tech industry.

5. Name: Emily Rodriguez

Location: Florida

Occupation: Nurse

Age: 45

Emily, a compassionate nurse in the Sunshine State of Florida, recognized the toll her demanding job took on her well-being. With a focus on nurturing her liver and gallbladder, she adopted a cleanse tailored to her high-stakes profession. Emily's journey showcased the vital role of healthcare professionals prioritizing self-care, inspiring her colleagues to consider holistic approaches to maintain their health.

6. Maria Gonzalez - Elementary School Teacher

Maria, a passionate elementary school teacher, chose to cleanse as a means of boosting her energy levels. Balancing a demanding job and caring for her students, Maria felt the need for a reset. Her cleanse included colorful salads, herbal teas, and daily walks in the school garden. The motivation behind her cleanse was to set a positive example for her students, teaching them the importance of nourishing the body and mind.

7. Dr. Ahmed Khan - Emergency Room Physician

For Dr. Ahmed Khan, an emergency room physician, the motivation for a cleanse was stress management. Dealing with high-pressure situations daily, Dr. Khan integrated mindfulness practices into his routine. His cleanse involved herbal supplements, yoga sessions, and regular breaks for deep breathing. The experience not only supported his liver health but also enhanced his ability to handle stressful situations with a calm and focused mind.

8. Sophie Williams - Marketing Executive

As a marketing executive navigating deadlines and creative challenges, Sophie Williams embarked on a cleanse to improve mental clarity. Her cleanse included nutrient-dense smoothies and intermittent fasting. Sophie found that detoxifying her body positively impacted her cognitive function, fostering innovative thinking and boosting her overall productivity in the fast-paced world of marketing.

9. Carlos Rodriguez - Construction Worker

Carlos Rodriguez, a hardworking construction worker, chose to cleanse to alleviate joint pain and fatigue. His physically demanding job required a holistic approach. Carlos incorporated anti-inflammatory foods into his diet and performed gentle stretching exercises. The cleanse not only supported his liver but also provided relief for his tired muscles, allowing him to continue his work with renewed vitality.

10. Alicia Chang - IT Professional

Alicia Chang, an IT professional, undertook a cleanse to address the sedentary nature of her job. Sitting at a desk for long hours, Alicia incorporated movement breaks, herbal teas, and a plant-based diet into her routine. The cleanse not only helped with digestion but also served as a reminder to prioritize self-care in a field known for long hours and demanding projects.

11. Eduardo Martinez - Small Business Owner

Eduardo Martinez, a small business owner, integrated a cleanse into his life to foster work-life balance. Juggling the responsibilities of entrepreneurship, Eduardo recognized the importance of maintaining good health. His cleanse included regular workouts, mindfulness practices, and a focus on hydration. The experience not only supported his liver and gallbladder health but also improved his overall well-being, positively influencing his business decisions.

Learn From Experiences, Challenges, and Triumphs

Learning from experiences, challenges, and triumphs holds particular relevance when considering a "Liver Gallbladder Cleanse." This holistic approach to well-being involves not only the physical aspect of cleansing but also the mental and emotional facets that come with undertaking such a journey.

Experiences:

In the context of a Liver Gallbladder Cleanse, individual experiences play a vital role in shaping the approach to the cleanse. Positive experiences, such as feeling increased energy levels, improved digestion, and enhanced well-being, serve as motivation to continue and refine the cleanse. Conversely, challenges encountered during the cleanse, such as adjusting to new dietary habits or facing detoxification symptoms, provide valuable insights into individual tolerances and areas for improvement.

Relating to Liver Gallbladder Cleanse: Positive experiences during a cleanse might include an individual feeling lighter, experiencing improved digestion, or noticing clearer skin. On the other hand, challenges might arise in adapting to a specific dietary protocol or dealing with detox symptoms such as headaches or fatigue. These experiences guide individuals in tailoring the cleanse to suit their unique needs and tolerances.

Challenges:

Challenges in the context of a Liver Gallbladder Cleanse are opportunities for growth and adaptation. For example, someone may face challenges in giving up certain foods or adjusting to a more plant-based diet. Overcoming these challenges provides insights into personal habits, triggers, and areas that may need more attention during the cleanse.

Relating to Liver Gallbladder Cleanse: A common challenge in a cleanse may involve reducing the intake of processed foods, sugar, and alcohol. Overcoming these challenges not only supports the cleanse process but also prompts a reevaluation of dietary choices for long-term well-being.

Triumphs:

Triumphs in a Liver Gallbladder Cleanse include achieving specific health goals, such as improved liver function, reduced inflammation, or weight management. Celebrating these triumphs reinforces positive behaviors and fosters a sense of accomplishment, motivating individuals to stay committed to their well-being journey.

Relating to Liver Gallbladder Cleanse: A triumph in a Liver Gallbladder Cleanse might be reflected in improved liver enzyme levels, a reduction in digestive discomfort, or achieving a weight loss goal. Acknowledging these triumphs encourages individuals to persist in their cleansing efforts and consider long-term lifestyle changes.

Reflection:

Reflection is a crucial aspect of a Liver Gallbladder Cleanse. Individuals may reflect on their dietary choices, stress levels, and overall lifestyle, identifying patterns that impact their liver and gallbladder health. Regular reflection provides an opportunity for adjustments and ensures that the cleanse remains tailored to the individual's evolving needs.

Relating to Liver Gallbladder Cleanse: Reflection might involve assessing the impact of specific foods on digestive comfort or recognizing the connection between stress levels and liver health. This self-awareness guides individuals in making informed choices that support their liver and gallbladder throughout the cleanse.

Adaptability:

Adaptability is key when undergoing a Liver Gallbladder Cleanse. As individuals learn from their experiences, navigate challenges, and celebrate triumphs, they become more adaptable in refining their approach to the cleanse. This adaptability ensures that the cleanse remains sustainable and tailored to individual needs.

Relating to Liver Gallbladder Cleanse: Adaptability may involve modifying the cleanse protocol based on individual responses, incorporating new detox support practices, or adjusting dietary choices to suit evolving preferences and goals.

Continuous Improvement:

Continuous improvement is inherent in the concept of a Liver Gallbladder Cleanse. As individuals learn and adapt, they continually refine their approach to achieve optimal results. This commitment to improvement is a lifelong journey that extends beyond the cleanse, influencing long-term lifestyle choices for sustained well-being.

Relating to Liver Gallbladder Cleanse: Continuous improvement in the context of a Liver Gallbladder

Cleanse may involve incorporating new liver-supporting foods, fine-tuning detox practices, and embracing a holistic approach to overall health that extends well beyond the cleanse period.

In conclusion, the principles of learning from experiences, challenges, and triumphs are integral to the success and sustainability of a Liver Gallbladder Cleanse. This approach ensures that the cleanse is not a rigid, one-size-fits-all process but a dynamic, personalized journey towards optimal liver and gallbladder health.

CHAPTER EIGHT
TROUBLESHOOTING THE CLEANSE: COMMON QUESTIONS AND EXPERT ANSWERS

Addressing Common Concerns About Liver-Gallbladder Cleansing

Liver-gallbladder cleansing has gained popularity as a holistic approach to supporting liver health and overall well-being. However, it is not uncommon for individuals to have concerns or questions about this process. Let's address some of the common concerns associated with liver-gallbladder cleansing:

---

1. Safety Concerns:

Concern:

- Is liver-gallbladder cleansing safe?

Response:

- Liver-gallbladder cleansing, when done with a mindful approach and under the guidance of a healthcare professional, is generally considered safe for most individuals. It's crucial to choose methods that are evidence-based and to avoid extreme or prolonged cleanses. If there are pre-existing health conditions, consulting with a healthcare provider is advisable.

Concern:

- Will I experience detox symptoms, and are they normal?

Response:

- It's not uncommon to experience mild detox symptoms such as headaches, fatigue, or changes in bowel habits during a cleanse. These symptoms are often temporary and indicate that the body is eliminating toxins. Staying hydrated, getting adequate rest, and gradually easing into the cleanse can help manage these symptoms.

Concern:

- Can liver-gallbladder cleansing intcrfcrc with medications?

Response:

- It's important to inform healthcare providers about any cleansing or dietary changes, especially if taking medications. Some herbs or supplements used in cleanses may interact with medications. A healthcare professional can provide guidance on how to safely incorporate a cleanse without compromising medication efficacy.

4. Nutrient Deficiency:

Concern:

- Will a cleanse lead to nutrient deficiencies?

Response:

- A well-balanced liver-gallbladder cleanse that includes a variety of nutrient-dense foods is unlikely to cause nutrient deficiencies. However, it's essential to monitor nutrient intake and, if needed, supplement appropriately. Working with a nutritionist or healthcare provider can help ensure that the cleanse is nutritionally sound.

---

5. Effectiveness:

Concern:

- How effective is liver-gallbladder cleansing?

Response:

- The effectiveness of a cleanse can vary among individuals. Some may experience improved energy, digestion, and overall well-being, while others may have more subtle benefits. The effectiveness depends on factors such as diet, lifestyle, and individual health conditions. It's essential to approach cleansing as part of a holistic lifestyle, incorporating long-term healthy habits.

Concern:

- How often should I cleanse my liver and gallbladder?

Response:

- The frequency of liver-gallbladder cleansing depends on individual health goals and needs. For some, an annual or semi-annual cleanse may be sufficient, while others may choose a more frequent approach. However, continuous cleansing without adequate breaks may not be necessary or beneficial. Consulting with a healthcare provider can help determine an appropriate schedule.

Concern:

- Can liver-gallbladder cleansing lead to dehydration?

Response:

- Proper hydration is crucial during any cleanse. While some methods may include increased fluid intake, it's essential to balance this with electrolytes. Drinking water, herbal teas, and incorporating hydrating foods like fruits and vegetables can help prevent dehydration. Monitoring urine color is a simple way to ensure adequate hydration.

Concern:

- Is liver-gallbladder cleansing safe during pregnancy or nursing?

Response:

- Pregnant or nursing individuals should avoid aggressive cleanses that may lead to nutrient deficiencies. Gentle, nourishing practices that support liver health, such as consuming a nutrient-rich diet, staying hydrated, and incorporating herbs safe during pregnancy, can be more suitable. Always consult with a healthcare provider before starting any cleanse during pregnancy or while nursing.

In conclusion, addressing concerns about liver-gallbladder cleansing involves approaching the process with mindfulness, seeking guidance from healthcare professionals, and ensuring that individual health needs are taken into account. A well-informed and balanced approach to liver-gallbladder cleansing can contribute to overall well-being when done responsibly and with consideration of individual health circumstances.

Expert Insights, Tips, and Troubleshooting Advice for Liver-Gallbladder Cleansing

Embarking on a liver-gallbladder cleanse can be a transformative journey for overall well-being. Here are expert insights, tips, and troubleshooting advice to ensure a safe and effective cleanse:

1. Consultation with Healthcare Professionals:

Insight:

- Before initiating a cleanse, consult with a healthcare professional, especially if you have pre-existing health conditions or are taking medications. They can provide personalized advice based on your health status.

Tips:

- Share your intentions to cleanse with your healthcare provider.

- Discuss any concerns, allergies, or sensitivities.

Troubleshooting:

- If you experience unexpected symptoms, consult your healthcare provider promptly.

- Adjust the cleanse based on their recommendations.

2. Hydration and Electrolyte Balance:

Insight:

- Proper hydration is essential during a cleanse, but maintaining electrolyte balance is equally important to prevent dehydration.

Tips:

- Drink plenty of water, herbal teas, and add electrolyte-rich foods like coconut water.

- Monitor urine color to gauge hydration levels.

Troubleshooting:

- If experiencing signs of dehydration (e.g., dizziness, dark urine), increase fluid intake and consider electrolyte supplements.

---

3. Mindful and Gradual Approach:

Insight:

- Adopt a mindful and gradual approach to cleansing. Abrupt changes may lead to detox symptoms and discomfort.

Tips:

- Ease into the cleanse by gradually reducing processed foods and caffeine.

- Introduce liver-supportive foods like leafy greens, beets, and berries.

Troubleshooting:

- If detox symptoms are overwhelming, consider slowing down the pace of the cleanse.

- Focus on nourishing foods and gentle detox practices.

4. Incorporate Liver-Supportive Herbs:

Insight:

- Certain herbs can support liver health and aid in the cleansing process.

Tips:

- Consider incorporating herbs like milk thistle, dandelion, and turmeric into your cleanse.

- Brew herbal teas with liver-cleansing properties.

Troubleshooting:

- If new herbs cause adverse reactions, discontinue use and consult with a healthcare professional.

- Adjust herb quantities based on individual tolerance.

5. Balanced Nutrition:

Insight:

- Maintain a balanced and nutrient-dense diet to support overall health and prevent nutrient deficiencies.

Tips:

- Include a variety of fruits, vegetables, whole grains, and lean proteins.

- Choose organic options when possible to minimize exposure to toxins.

Troubleshooting:

- If concerns about nutrient deficiencies arise, consult with a nutritionist for personalized advice.

- Monitor energy levels and adjust dietary choices accordingly.

---

6. Mind-Body Practices:

Insight:

- Incorporate mind-body practices to manage stress, which can impact liver health.

Tips:

- Practice meditation, deep breathing, or yoga to reduce stress levels.

- Ensure adequate sleep to support the body's natural detoxification processes.

Troubleshooting:

- If stress levels are high, prioritize relaxation practices.

- Consider professional guidance for stress management techniques.

---

7. Monitoring Detox Symptoms:

Insight:

- Expect mild detox symptoms, but monitor for signs of excessive discomfort.

Tips:

- Common detox symptoms include headaches, fatigue, and changes in bowel habits.

- Keep a journal to track symptoms and overall well-being.

Troubleshooting:

- If detox symptoms are severe or prolonged, consult with a healthcare professional.

- Adjust the cleanse based on individual tolerance and needs.

8. Post-Cleanse Transition:

Insight:

- Gradually transition back to a regular diet post-cleanse to avoid digestive discomfort.

Tips:

- Introduce foods gradually, starting with easily digestible options.

- Continue to prioritize liver-supportive foods in your regular diet.

Troubleshooting:

- If digestive issues persist, consult with a nutritionist or healthcare provider for guidance.

- Adjust the pace of reintroducing foods based on individual responses.

In summary, approaching a liver-gallbladder cleanse with expert insights, thoughtful tips, and troubleshooting advice enhances the likelihood of a successful and positive experience. Individualize your cleanse, listen to your body, and seek professional guidance when needed to optimize the benefits of the cleansing process.

CHAPTER NINE
YOUR ROADMAP TO SUSTAINABLE WELLNESS: POST-CLEANSE MAINTENANCE AND BEYOND

Navigating The Post-Cleanse Phase with A Sustainable Wellness Roadmap

Completing a liver-gallbladder cleanse is a significant accomplishment, and the post-cleanse phase is a crucial time to integrate sustainable practices for ongoing well-being. Here's a roadmap to guide you through this phase and maintain a healthy and balanced lifestyle:

1. Gradual Reintroduction of Foods:

Approach:

- Gradually reintroduce a diverse range of foods to avoid digestive discomfort.
- Focus on nutrient-dense options like fruits, vegetables, whole grains, and lean proteins.

Sustainable Tip:

- Embrace a varied and balanced diet to provide essential nutrients for overall health.
- Incorporate seasonal and locally sourced foods when possible.

2. Maintain Hydration and Detox Support:

Approach:

- Continue prioritizing hydration with water, herbal teas, and electrolyte-rich beverages.

- Integrate liver-supportive herbs and foods into your regular diet.

Sustainable Tip:

- Make hydration a daily habit, aiming for at least eight glasses of water per day.

- Include herbs like dandelion and turmeric in meals for ongoing liver support.

3. Mindful Eating Practices:

Approach:

- Practice mindful eating to foster a healthy relationship with food.

- Pay attention to hunger and fullness cues, savoring each bite.

Sustainable Tip:

- Avoid distractions while eating, such as watching TV or using electronic devices.

- Express gratitude for the nourishment your food provides.

4. Regular Exercise Routine:

Approach:

- Establish a regular exercise routine that includes a mix of cardiovascular, strength, and flexibility exercises.

- Choose activities you enjoy to make exercise a sustainable part of your lifestyle.

Sustainable Tip:

- Aim for at least 150 minutes of moderate-intensity exercise per week.

- Incorporate activities like walking, cycling, or dancing into your routine.

5. Stress Management Techniques:

Approach:

- Continue incorporating stress management techniques like meditation, deep breathing, or yoga.

- Prioritize adequate sleep to support overall well-being.

Sustainable Tip:

- Schedule regular moments of relaxation, even on busy days.

- Create a bedtime routine to promote quality sleep.

6. Regular Health Check-ups:

Approach:

- Schedule regular health check-ups and screenings to monitor overall health.

- Discuss with healthcare providers any concerns or changes in well-being.

Sustainable Tip:

- Keep a health journal to track symptoms, energy levels, and overall mood.

- Stay proactive in addressing health issues and seeking professional advice.

Approach:

- Explore holistic wellness practices that resonate with you, such as acupuncture, massage, or aromatherapy.
- Consider integrating mind-body practices like tai chi or qigong.

Sustainable Tip:

- Choose practices that align with your lifestyle and bring you joy.
- Regularly engage in activities that promote relaxation and self-care.

Approach:

- Cultivate a supportive community of friends, family, or like-minded individuals.
- Share your wellness journey and seek encouragement from those around you.

Sustainable Tip:

- Join local or online communities focused on health and well-being.
- Participate in activities or events that foster connections and shared interests.

By embracing this sustainable wellness roadmap, you can transition smoothly into the post-cleanse phase and cultivate habits that contribute to your long-term health and vitality. Remember that wellness is an ongoing journey, and small, consistent steps can lead to significant and lasting improvements in your overall well-being.

Daily Habits and Practices for Enduring Liver and Gallbladder Health

Maintaining the health of your liver and gallbladder is crucial for overall well-being. Incorporating daily habits and practices can support these vital organs and promote long-term health. Here's a guide to enduring liver and gallbladder health:

1. Hydration:

Daily Habit:

- Start your day with a glass of water and stay hydrated throughout the day.
- Include herbal teas known for liver support, such as dandelion or milk thistle tea.

Practice:

- Carry a reusable water bottle to ensure you can hydrate wherever you go.
- Infuse water with lemon or cucumber for added flavor and detox benefits.

2. Balanced Nutrition:

Daily Habit:

- Emphasize a balanced diet rich in fruits, vegetables, whole grains, and lean proteins.
- Choose foods high in antioxidants, like berries and leafy greens, to support liver health.

Practice:

- Plan your meals to include a variety of colors and nutrients.

- Minimize processed foods, saturated fats, and added sugars in your diet.

3. Herbs and Supplements:

Daily Habit:

- Consider incorporating liver-supportive herbs like turmeric, ginger, and artichoke into your meals.

- Take high-quality supplements, such as omega-3 fatty acids, if needed.

Practice:

- Consult with a healthcare professional before adding new herbs or supplements to your routine.

- Ensure the quality and authenticity of any herbal products you use.

4. Mindful Eating:

Daily Habit:

- Practice mindful eating by savoring each bite and paying attention to hunger and fullness cues.

- Eat smaller, more frequent meals throughout the day to support digestion.

Practice:

- Avoid distractions like television or smartphones during meals.

- Chew your food thoroughly to aid in digestion.

5. Regular Exercise:

Daily Habit:

- Establish a daily exercise routine that includes both aerobic and strength-training exercises.
- Aim for at least 30 minutes of moderate-intensity exercise most days of the week.

Practice:

- Find activities you enjoy to make exercise a sustainable part of your routine.
- Incorporate movement into your day, such as taking the stairs or going for a walk.

6. Stress Management:

Daily Habit:

- Incorporate stress management techniques like meditation, deep breathing, or yoga into your daily routine.
- Prioritize adequate sleep, aiming for 7-8 hours per night.

Practice:

- Create a calming bedtime routine to signal to your body that it's time to wind down.
- Schedule regular breaks during the day to reset and relax.

7. Limit Alcohol Consumption:

Daily Habit:

- If you consume alcohol, do so in moderation. Limit the amount and frequency of alcohol intake.

- Consider alcohol-free days during the week to give your liver a break.

Practice:

- Be mindful of portion sizes and choose lower-alcohol options when available.

- Alternate alcoholic beverages with water to stay hydrated.

8. Regular Health Check-ups:

Daily Habit:

- Schedule regular health check-ups and screenings to monitor liver and overall health.

- Be proactive in addressing any health concerns with your healthcare provider.

Practice:

- Keep track of any changes in your body or well-being and discuss them during check-ups.

- Share your lifestyle choices and habits with your healthcare provider for personalized advice.

Daily Habit:

- Cultivate a positive mindset by expressing gratitude and focusing on positive aspects of your life.

- Surround yourself with a supportive community that uplifts and encourages you.

Practice:

- Practice self-compassion and avoid harsh self-criticism.

- Engage in activities that bring you joy and contribute to a positive outlook.

Incorporating these daily habits and practices into your routine can contribute to enduring liver and gallbladder health. Remember that consistency is key, and making small, sustainable changes over time can have a significant impact on your overall well-being.

CONCLUSION

Prioritizing the health of your liver and gallbladder through mindful daily habits and practices is a proactive and sustainable approach to overall well-being. The interconnected nature of nutrition, hydration, exercise, stress management, and positive mindset plays a vital role in supporting these essential organs.

By adopting a balanced and nutrient-dense diet, staying hydrated, incorporating liver-supportive herbs, and engaging in regular physical activity, you provide your body with the tools it needs for optimal function. Mindful practices such as stress management, adequate sleep, and cultivating a positive mindset contribute not only to liver and gallbladder health but to holistic wellness.

Remember that wellness is a journey, and small, consistent efforts compound over time. Regular health check-ups, consultation with healthcare professionals, and staying attuned to your body's signals are crucial aspects of maintaining enduring liver and gallbladder health.

Ultimately, by integrating these practices into your daily life, you empower yourself to take charge of your health and promote a resilient foundation for a fulfilling and vibrant life. The commitment to these habits reflects a holistic understanding of well-being, recognizing the profound impact of lifestyle choices on the intricate balance of body and mind. Here's to a journey of sustained health, vitality, and overall wellness.